Table of Contents

INTRODUCTION

According to recent research, at least one in three Alzheimer's disease cases worldwide is preventable. One of the closest things we know of to a natural Alzheimer's treatment is a healthy, anti-inflammatory diet. That's because foods like vegetables, fruit, nuts and fish are high in antioxidants, healthy fats and other phytochemicals that help protect the brain from disease. According to many studies, the Mediterranean and DASH diets have the ability to slow aging and cognitive decline in older adults. For years, both of these diets have been considered two of the best for protecting against diseases related to aging, inflammation and oxidative stress. For example, many studies have found that the Mediterranean diet and DASH diet can be helpful for lowering adults' risk for high blood pressure, high cholesterol, cardiovascular disease, diabetes, obesity, PCOS and a number of age-related neurological conditions. Given the anti-aging effects that these two diets have to offer, it's no surprise that elements of both are now being combined in order to boost mental/cognitive health in those who are most susceptible.

The MIND diet stands for Mediterranean-DASH Intervention for Neurodegenerative Delay. This diet combines principles from two other well-known diets: the Mediterranean diet and the DASH (Dietary Approaches to Stop Hypertension) diet. The Mediterranean diet is inspired by the traditional eating habits of those in Mediterranean countries. The DASH diet was developed as a result of clinical trials funded by the National Heart, Lung and Blood Institute (NHLBI). In the MIND diet, parts of these diets have been combined with a new goal: reduce dementia and a decline in brain health that usually occurs as we age. Specifically, the MIND diet differs from the Mediterranean and DASH diets in a few ways: It emphasizes berries, due to their antioxidant properties, over other fruits and recommends eating fish at least once per week. It also highlights the difference between green, leafy vegetables, which are rich in many nutrients and thought to reduce the risk of CVD and cognitive decline, and "other vegetables." The MIND diet argues that both green leafy vegetables and other vegetables are essential.

Both the Mediterranean and DASH diets have been researched thoroughly and are associated with lower blood pressure, a decreased risk of cardiovascular disease and Type 2 diabetes. In contrast, there are only a handful of epidemiological studies examining the MIND diet's effect on brain health and cognitive function. So far, the results have shown the MIND diet to be associated with slowing cognitive decline and a reduced risk for Alzheimer's disease. One of the theories behind its health benefits is that foods emphasized on the MIND diet are rich in antioxidants, which can reduce oxidative stress. Oxidative stress is defined as an imbalance between the production of free radicals and antioxidant defenses, and prolonged exposure can cause cell damage – particularly to the brain. Additionally, because the MIND diet is a combination of the Mediterranean diet and DASH diet, it's thought to have a similar effect on improving heart health and reducing the risk of CVD and diabetes, both of which are risk factors for Alzheimer's disease.

The MIND diet was created to prevent dementia and loss of brain activities with age. Coincidently, the name of the

MIND diet implies a diet designed to have a healthy mind and reduce the risk of Alzheimer's disease. MIND diet combines the Mediterranean diet and the DASH diet to form a new dietary plan that is meant to improve brain health. The MIND diet involves the intake of plant-based foods and avoiding the intake of animal products and foods which have high quantities of saturated fats. Although the MIND diet – in conjunction with other healthy habits like regular exercise, not smoking and getting adequate sleep – may have an effect on cognition, many other factors impact the development of Alzheimer's disease and presently, there is no cure for it.

CHAPTER ONE

The Basics of the MIND Diet

Now that people know which healthy foods to include in their diets, it is time to look at how those trying to follow the MIND diet can stick to it. Some of the key points to keep in mind include:

- Vary the Recipes: At the beginning of the diet, it might be hard to stick to the MIND method's restrictions. At the same time, getting creative is always helpful. Take a look at the diet and see what tastes good. Then, find creative recipes to switch up the tastes. This will prevent the diet from seeming monotonous.

- Set Realistic Expectations: Nobody is going to expect someone to switch up their diet overnight. Therefore, setting realistic goals and easing into the diet is an excellent place to start. Try to be flexible and remove one food from the diet at a time. Then, over time, switching to the MIND diet won't seem like such a significant shift.

- Keep Bad Foods Out of the Home: Finally, try to keep out foods that are not on the healthy side of the diet by not having them in the house. This will remove temptation. Furthermore, try to carry healthy snacks to munch on throughout the day. This can help everyone stick to the MIND diet more easily.

By remembering the MIND diet's real motivation, everyone will be able to use these tips to stick to healthy foods and avoid bad ones. Then, everyone can enjoy the neuroprotective benefits of the MIND diet!

What Is the MIND Diet?

MIND stands for the Mediterranean-DASH Intervention for Neurodegenerative Delay. The MIND diet aims to reduce dementia and the decline in brain health that often occurs as people get older. It combines aspects of two very popular diets, the Mediterranean diet and the Dietary Approaches to Stop Hypertension (DASH) diet. Many experts regard the Mediterranean and DASH diets as some of the healthiest. Research has shown they can lower blood pressure and reduce the risk of heart disease, diabetes and several other diseases. But researchers wanted to create a diet specifically to help improve brain function and prevent dementia. To do this, they combined foods from the Mediterranean and DASH diets that had been shown to benefit brain health.

For example, both the Mediterranean and DASH diets recommend eating a lot of fruit. Fruit intake has not been correlated with improved brain function, but eating berries has been. Thus, the MIND diet encourages its followers to eat berries, but does not emphasize consuming fruit in general. Currently, there are no set guidelines for how to follow the MIND diet. Simply eat more of the 10 foods the diet encourages you to eat, and eat less of the five foods the diet recommends you limit.

The MIND diet is a fusion of two diets considered to be among the most healthy, the Mediterranean diet and the DASH diet. The Mediterranean diet is one of the most popular and widely researched ways of eating. It emphasizes vegetables, fruits, nuts, fish, olive oil, and red wine. The DASH diet (Dietary Approaches to Stop Hypertension) was developed by the US National Heart,

Lung, and Blood Institute for treating high blood pressure. It also centers around eating whole grains, vegetables, and fruits, but, unlike the Mediterranean diet, is a low-sodium diet. The MIND diet — short for the Mediterranean-Dash Intervention for Neurodegenerative Delay diet — is a healthy eating plan that has the goal of lowering your risk for cognitive disorders, like Alzheimer's disease and dementia.

The MIND diet (also sometimes called the Med-DASH plan) was first introduced in 2016. It is based on principles of both the Mediterranean diet and the DASH diet (which stands for Dietary Approaches to Stop Hypertension, or in other words high blood pressure diet). The DASH diet and Mediterranean diet have both been named at one time the "#1 best overall diet" in the United States by U.S. News and World Report. What does the MIND diet consist of? Just like the two eating plans it combines, the MIND diet includes lots of "brain foods" that boost focus and memory — such as leafy greens, berries, nuts, olive oil and fatty fish. Examples of MIND diet recipes might include salmon cooked in olive oil with wilted greens and quinoa or oatmeal topped with almonds and blueberries.

How Does the MIND Diet Work?

To follow the MIND diet effectively, it is essential to take a closer look at how it works. The MIND diet is much easier to follow than other diets, including the Mediterranean diet, which means that people should have an easier time sticking to it. In general, the diet has fifteen separate components. Ten food groups have been dubbed as "brain-healthy." These include:

- Whole grains
- Fish
- Poultry
- Olive oil
- Wine
- Green leafy vegetables
- Other vegetables
- Nuts
- Berries
- Beans

In addition to the ten healthy food groups above, there are also five unhealthy food groups. These include:

- Fried or fast food
- Red meats
- Butter and stick margarine
- Cheese
- Pastries and sweets

Based on the information above, it should be clear that the MIND diet's goal is to stick to the healthy food groups at the top of the list and avoid the unhealthy food groups as much as possible. In general, those who are looking to follow the MIND diet will follow these instructions:

- It is essential to eat at least three servings of whole grains, at least one salad, and at least one other vegetable every day.
- Some people might be glad to hear that a glass of wine per day is also included in this diet.
- Every other day, people should try to snack on nuts and eat a helping of beans.
- Twice per week, people should try to eat berries.

- Once per week, those following the MIND diet should eat one serving of fish.

It is also important to limit unhealthy food to less than one serving per week to lower the risk of Alzheimer's disease.

How Healthy is the MIND Diet?

Both the Mediterranean and DASH diets are considered extremely healthy. The former is linked to lower risk of death from heart disease and cancer as well as to improvements in brain function and lower rates of chronic disease and offers protection from Alzheimer's disease. In addition to helping lower blood pressure, the DASH diet can help reduce blood levels of homocysteine, a toxic amino acid. People with high blood levels of homocysteine have twice the normal risk of developing Alzheimer's disease.

How Popular Is It?

Although the MIND diet has received much favorable publicity, the extent of its popularity is unknown. The Alzheimer's Association has featured it on its website, and a U.S. News and World Report panel of experts ranked it fourth healthiest OF 41 diets reviewed as well as the fourth easiest diet to follow, the fourth best heart healthy diet and the fourth best for healthy eating generally. An ongoing three-year study of the MIND diet at Rush University and the Harvard T.H. Chan School of Public Health will examine its effects on cognitive decline and brain health in a group of 600 participants between the ages of 65 and 84 who have a family history (but no personal history) of dementia, are overweight or obese and have poor eating habits.

General Principles of The MIND Diet

The MIND diet, which is known as the Mediterranean-DASH Intervention for Neurodegenerative Delay, had been developed by the late Martha Clare Morris, a nutritional epidemiologist of that time at Rush University Medical Center. Different research has revealed that the MIND Diet decreased the risk of Alzheimer's diseases by 35%. The MIND diet also plays a protective role against Parkinson's disease. The MIND diet is a blend of two proven healthy diets. It also boosts brain power. The MIND diet is all about eating at least three servings of whole grains, a salad, and a vegetable. Also, you can drink a glass of wine. When you are following the MIND diet, you can eat snacks and nuts on most days along with a half cup of beans.

Moreover, when you are on the MIND diet, you can have poultry at least two times a week. Also, you can have a half-cup serving of berries. With the MIND diet, you can have a balanced proportion of all nutrients. So, it has become popular as one of the healthiest eating patterns of all time. Since there are no treatments to reverse Alzheimer's disease or other forms of dementia, we need strategies to help prevent them. The MIND diet with its focus on the effects of foods on brain health may be one such strategy.

How the MIND Diet Can Help Reduce Dementia and Alzheimer's Risk

The MIND diet is valued most for its ability to support brain function and reduce neurodegeneration (the progressive loss of structure or function of neurons, including death of neurons). A 2015 study published in Alzheimer's and Dementia (the journal of the Alzheimer's Association) that followed over 900 adults found that those who ate in a similar way to the MIND diet had a 53 percent lower risk of developing Alzheimer's disease compared to the adults who ate very differently than the MIND diet. Another positive finding was that adults didn't have to stick to the MIND diet perfectly or be very strict with themselves to see real benefits. Even those who only "moderately" followed the MIND diet were found to have about a 35 percent reduced risk for Alzheimer's disease, on average. Another study found that the "difference in decline rates for being in the top tertile of MIND diet scores versus the lowest was equivalent to being 7.5 years younger in age." This suggests that the MIND diet substantially slows cognitive decline with age. The brain is very susceptible to the effects of oxidative stress, especially as someone ages. This is partially responsible for loss of memory, learning capacity, mood stabilization, etc. What is one food that fights dementia and protects the aging brain? There are actually a number of foods that have been shown to help support memory and brain function, especially those high in protective antioxidants, such as strawberries and blueberries (which contain flavonoids like anthocyanidins), olive oil, dark chocolate, and green tea (which contain polyphenols). For example, according to the large study called the Nurse's Healthy Study, anthocyanidins and flavonoids found in plant foods like berries are associated with slower rates of cognitive decline. This particular study found that frequent berry consumption may help delay cognitive aging by up to 2.5 years. There's good evidence that what you eat can make a difference in your risk of cognitive decline and dementia, including Alzheimer's disease. Here's what to do about it. The research is in: Eating certain foods (and avoiding others) has been shown to slow brain aging by 7.5 years, and lessen the chances of developing Alzheimer's disease. This isn't some trendy diet of the moment. Born as a hybrid of two existing eating styles with decades of research at their backs — the DASH diet and Mediterranean diet — university researchers developed the MIND diet to emphasize foods that impact brain health.

Here's what that looks like:

Load up on vegetables

Just like Mom always told you: Eat your vegetables. But unique to the MIND diet, researchers found that green leafy ones like kale, collards, spinach or lettuce were specifically shown to lower the risk of dementia and cognitive decline. Greens are packed with nutrients linked to better brain health like folate, vitamin E, carotenoids and flavonoids. And one serving a day has been shown to slow brain aging. To max out your veggie score, aim to eat at least six servings a week of greens. Then round it out with at least one serving of other vegetables a day.

Make berries your sweet treat

Nothing against the apple a day, but when scientists reviewed the research on diet and brain health, one type of fruit soared above the rest: berries. In a 20-year study of over 16,000 older adults, those who ate the most blueberries and strawberries had the slowest rates of cognitive decline. Researchers credit the high levels of flavonoids in berries with the benefit. Treat yourself to two or more berry servings a week for peak brain health.

Nuts may be high in calories and fat, but they're packed with fat-soluble vitamin E, known for its brain-protective qualities. Grab a handful at least five times a week instead of processed snacks like chips or pastries. Check the list of ingredients and opt for the dry-roasted or raw, unsalted kind without extra sodium, sweeteners or oils. (Hint: No-stir peanut butters have stuff added.)

Another Mediterranean diet staple that has a home in the MIND diet is olive oil. Researchers recommend using it as your primary cooking oil, and avoiding butter and margarine. New to olive oil? Look for "extra virgin" olive oil (skip anything labeled "light") and choose a bottle that's opaque or dark glass since light causes it to go bad faster.

Brain-healthy eating encourages consuming meat sparingly (red meat makes an appearance fewer than four times a week in the ideal MIND diet). Beans, lentils and soybeans, which pack protein and fiber, make a worthy substitute. They'll keep you full and are rich in B vitamins, which are important for brain health. In one study analyzing the diets of older adults, those who had the lowest intakes of legumes had greater cognitive decline than those who ate more.

Have fish once a week

Constantly forgetting the name of that person you just met? Adults age 65 and older who ate fish once a week or more scored better on memory tests and tricky number games than those who had seafood less often. But if fish isn't your favorite, there's good news: MIND diet researchers couldn't find proof that having it more than once a week added extra benefits for the brain.

Feel free to savor a glass of wine

While too much alcohol is unquestionably harmful to the brain and overall health, studies suggest that light to moderate drinking may lower the risk of dementia. And it may delay the onset of Alzheimer's by two to three years. One possible reason: Alcohol seems to help blood flow, making it less sticky and less prone to potentially harmful clotting. Given the risks of alcohol, it's probably not a good idea to start drinking it just for the possible brain benefit. But if you enjoy a glass of wine with dinner, you can continue the habit on the MIND diet.

Researchers believe that high-antioxidant foods included in the MIND diet positively impact learning, memory and cognition. Here are some of the reasons why:

- They protect aging neurons against the negative impact of stress-related cellular signals, increasing the capacity of neurons to maintain proper functioning during aging.

- A key component of the MIND diet, green leafy vegetables like kale or spinach, are believed to protect the brain because they contain high levels of compounds that fight oxidative stress. Antioxidants found in dark leafy greens include lutein, zeaxanthin, phenols and flavonoids.

- The MIND diet encourages consumption of healthy fats that fuel the brain, such as fish like salmon and certain nuts/seeds like walnuts or flaxseed that contain omega-3 fatty acids. Omega-3s have anti-inflammatory properties that support the neurological and immune systems, and healthy fats in general (including some cholesterol) are important for brain health because they help form neuron connections and also help manage levels of blood glucose (sugar).

- Foods that are brightly colored — like carrots, tomatoes, kale and sweet potatoes, which all contain carotenoid antioxidants — may help prevent the formation of beta-amyloid plaques in the brain. Beta-amyloids are proteins that can build up in the brain, forming plaque deposits and neurofibrillary tangles that are thought to contribute to the degradation of the nerve cells. Production and accumulation of beta-amyloids in the brain are now believed to be a major contributing factor to Alzheimer's disease.

How does the MIND diet help brain health?

Adults who follow the MIND diet have a slower overall rate of cognitive decline, which researchers say is equivalent to 7.5 years of younger age. This is due to the nutritious combination of foods promoted on the diet, which help reduce inflammation and preserve white matter in the brain. These aspects are linked to stronger cognitive benefits. The MIND diet is rich in nutrients such as folate, vitamin E, lutein-zeaxanthin, and flavonoids. These nutrients are known for their anti-inflammatory, antioxidant, and pro-cognition properties.

For example, green leafy vegetables and nuts contain vitamin E, an antioxidant that protects neurons from damage related to oxidative stress caused by free radicals. And berries help reverse neuronal aging by reducing oxidative stress. All of the foods on the MIND diet work synergistically to protect brain health. "The MIND diet is developed based on the Mediterranean and DASH diets but with modifications that emphasize foods for brain health, such as green leafy vegetables and berries. These foods are sources of vitamin E, carotenoids, and flavonoids, which are nutrients related to the risk of dementia,"

Foods to Eat

What can you eat on the MIND diet? The MIND diet emphasizes these healthy food groups:

- Vegetables, especially leafy greens like spinach, kale, etc.

- All other fresh vegetables are also included, such as cruciferous veggies like broccoli, Brussels sprouts, peppers, tomatoes, carrots, mushrooms, green beans, etc.

- Fresh fruit, especially all types of berries, including strawberries, blueberries, raspberries, blackberries, cherries, cranberries, etc.

- Nuts and seeds, such as walnuts, almonds, chia seeds and flaxseeds

- Beans and legumes, such as chickpeas, black beans, lentils, etc.

- 100 percent whole grains, such as oatmeal, quinoa, brown rice, barley, farro, 100 percent whole-wheat breads, etc.

- Fish, particularly wild-caught, fatty fish like like salmon, sardines, halibut, trout, tuna and mackerel, which are the best sources of omega-3 fats

- Lean meats like poultry, ideally that are pasture-raised and not breaded or fried
- Olive oil, which is used as the "main cooking oil" and can also be drizzled over salad, veggies, etc.

In addition to the foods above, the MIND diet allows room for about one glass of wine per day (ideally red wine, which is higher in the antioxidant called resveratrol), as well as treats like sweets in moderation. Are eggs allowed on the MIND diet? What about the MIND diet and dairy? Eggs are not specifically mentioned in the book "The MIND Diet," however many experts believe that eggs can be included in a healthy, balanced eating plan that supports brain health. That's because eggs are capable of supporting cognition, according to certain studies. They are nutrient-dense and a great source of B vitamins, choline, carotenoids like lutein and more. Eggs are also versatile, inexpensive, and a good source of healthy fats and protein. Dairy is another food group that is not discussed in great length in the MIND diet book. It's recommended that full-fat dairy products be limited to small quantities, such as one ounce of cheese one to two times per week. Many health authorities recommend consuming fermented dairy products, such as unsweetened yogurt or kefir, due to their beneficial supply of probiotics, minerals like calcium and many other nutrients. Dairy foods are also included in the Mediterranean diet, and low-fat dairy products are encouraged on the DASH diet.

Foods to Avoid

Now that you know which foods to eat on the MIND diet, let's talk about foods you want to limit. Foods to avoid on the MIND diet include:

- Most types of red meat, such as beef, pork and lamb — it's recommended that red meat be consumed no more than one to three times per week

- Butter and margarine (olive oil is encouraged instead)

- Cheese/full-fat dairy products

- Sugary snacks/sweets and sweetened beverages, including soda, ice cream, cookies, brownies, donuts, candy, etc.

- Fast foods, fried foods and packaged foods
- Any food that contains trans fats or hydrogenated fats and most foods with saturated fat

Many of these are known to be foods that raise your Alzheimer's risk. Regarding whether saturated fat should be limited, this remains a controversial topic. There's some evidence that high intake of saturated fat and trans fats may increase the risk for neurological conditions. However, overall findings about fat intake and risk for dementia/Alzheimer's have not been consistent. Certain studies have also found that intakes of total fat, animal fat and dietary cholesterol are not associated with Alzheimer's disease risk. It's recommended that you limit these less favorable foods on the MIND diet to these servings per week:

- Sweets — less than 3–5 servings per week.
- Butter and Margarine — Up to 1 tablespoon per day.
- Red Meat — Less than 3–4 servings per week.
- Whole Fat Cheese —Up to several servings per week or less.

- Fried Fast Foods — Less than 1 serving per week.

The MIND diet highlights the need to consume 1 serving of fish weekly, primarily for its omega-3 content. But some fish species can be high in contaminants such as mercury that can affect the nervous system and cognition. In one analysis, mercury had subtle effects on the developing nervous systems of newborns. Pregnant or breastfeeding women, as well as those planning to become pregnant, and very young children should avoid fish high in mercury (such as shark, swordfish, king mackerel, tuna, and golden bass).

The MIND diet highlights foods like wheat, legumes, and vegetables, including nightshades. All these foods may be problematic for some people. People with food allergies, chronic food sensitivities, lectin sensitivity, or autoimmune disorders may need to modify this diet to align with their specific needs and health status. Work with your doctor to develop the ideal diet for your health needs.

MIND Diet Meal Plan

The focus of the MIND diet is whole foods that are nutrient-dense. The best nutrient-dense foods are minimally processed, additive-free, ideally organic and often plant-based/vegetarian. The MIND eating plan is overall relatively low in total fat, especially saturated fat and cholesterol for the most part, and includes lots of fiber from fruits, vegetables and whole grains. As part of the MIND diet eating plan, incorporate the foods below, which are high in carotenoids, flavonoids and other phytochemicals, into as many meals as possible:

- Berries
- Pomegranate
- Acai
- Green tea and other teas, plus coffee
- Currants
- Tart cherry juice
- Dark cocoa
- Winter squash or butternut squash

- Carrots and carrot juice

- Sweet potato

- Tomatoes

- Onions

- Artichokes

- Pumpkin

- Spinach

- Plantains

- Kale

- Collard/turnip greens

- Citrus fruits (grapefruit, oranges and tangerines)

- Cantaloupe

- Red peppers

- Papaya

- Red wine

Aim to have these number of servings of the healthy MIND diet food groups listed above:

- Several servings of vegetables per day, especially leafy greens, which should ideally be eaten daily.

- Berries at least several times per week (aim for 4–5 weekly servings).

- Fatty fish 2–3 times per week.

- Poultry 2 or more times per week.

- At least several servings of nuts and beans/legumes per week (aim for 3–5 weekly servings).

- Whole grains on a regular basis, up to several servings per day.

- Olive oil just about daily, used as the main cooking oil and source of fat.

Here are ideas for making healthy MIND diet recipes:

- Berry green smoothies made with superfoods like spinach, blueberries, flaxseeds and almond milk.

- Salmon and kale salad with pomegranates, almonds, sliced oranges and fennel.

- Roasted red pepper chicken with sweet potatoes and broccoli drizzled with olive oil.

- Hummus served with eggplant, olive oil, roasted red peppers and whole grain pita.

Is it possible to follow a vegetarian MIND diet? Yes, you can stick to the MIND diet if you're vegetarian by getting protein from beans, legumes, whole grains, nuts, seeds and perhaps fish if you consume fish.

MIND Diet vs. Mediterranean Diet vs. Keto Diet

Because the MIND diet is based partially on the Mediterranean diet, the two have many things in common, such as emphasis on eating lots of plant foods, making olive oil and nuts the primary sources of fat, and having wine in moderation. What are some differences among these two diets? The MIND diet puts added emphasis on veggies like dark leafy greens, fruits like berries, beans, fish and poultry. It also limits dairy, which is included in both the Mediterranean diet and DASH diet. Overall, there is not much of a difference between the two plans, however many associate the Mediterranean diet with more ethnic foods like hummus, olives, whole wheat pita, tabouli, etc. The MIND diet is a bit more inclusive and puts equal value on different whole grains like brown rice, oats, legumes, etc.

While both have been shown to have anti-inflammatory effects and support weight loss, the MIND diet and ketogenic diet are considerably different. The keto diet is a high-fat, low-carb diet, while the MIND diet is basically the opposite: a higher-carb, high-fiber diet that includes moderate amounts of mostly unsaturated fats.

Some major differences between the two:
- The keto diet excludes all whole grains, fruit (with the exception of about 1/4 berries per day), legumes/beans (with the exception of about 1/4 berries per day) and any added sugar.
- It also emphasizes high consumption of healthy fats, which provide about 75 percent or more of calories, from foods like coconut oil, butter, ghee, olive oil, eggs, nuts, avocado and fattier cuts of meat.
- The MIND diet may be a better option to follow long -term, but the keto diet is more likely to lead to substantial weight loss, often quickly.

There are not many risks involved with the MIND diet, although it's best to tell your doctor about any major dietary changes you plan to make if you're currently being treated for a chronic condition. If you choose to follow the MIND diet meal plan, remember that you don't need to adhere to the diet perfectly to improve your health, so try to take a long-term approach to sticking with the diet. Of course, in addition to following a nutrient-dense diet to protect your brain, it's also wise to reduce your risk for cognitive disorders by avoiding the "main seven risk factors for Alzheimer's disease," which include:

- Diabetes
- Mid-life hypertension
- Mid-life obesity
- Physical inactivity
- Depression
- Smoking
- Low educational attainment

Making meals for the MIND diet doesn't have to be complicated. Center your meals around the 10 foods and food groups that are encouraged on the diet, and try to stay away from the five foods that need to be limited. Here's a seven-day meal plan to get you started:

Monday

- Breakfast: Greek yogurt with raspberries, topped with sliced almonds.
- Lunch: Mediterranean salad with olive-oil-based dressing, grilled chicken, whole-wheat pita.
- Dinner: Burrito bowl with brown rice, black beans, fajita vegetables, grilled chicken, salsa and guacamole.

Tuesday

- Breakfast: Wheat toast with almond butter, scrambled eggs.
- Lunch: Grilled chicken sandwich, blackberries, carrots.
- Dinner: Grilled salmon, side salad with olive-oil-based dressing, brown rice.

Wednesday

- Breakfast: Steel-cut oatmeal with strawberries, hard-boiled eggs.

- Lunch: Mexican-style salad with mixed greens, black beans, red onion, corn, grilled chicken and olive-oil-based dressing.

- Dinner: Chicken and vegetable stir-fry, brown rice.

Thursday

- Breakfast: Greek yogurt with peanut butter and banana.

- Lunch: Baked trout, collard greens, black-eyed peas.

- Dinner: Whole-wheat spaghetti with turkey meatballs and marinara sauce, side salad with olive-oil-based dressing.

Friday

- Breakfast: Wheat toast with avocado, omelet with peppers and onions.

- Lunch: Chili made with ground turkey.

- Dinner: Greek-seasoned baked chicken, oven-roasted potatoes, side salad, wheat dinner roll.

Saturday

- Breakfast: Overnight oats with strawberries.
- Lunch: Fish tacos on whole wheat tortillas, brown rice, pinto beans.
- Dinner: Chicken gyro on whole-wheat pita, cucumber and tomato salad.

Sunday

- Breakfast: Spinach frittata, sliced apple and peanut butter.
- Lunch: Tuna salad sandwich on wheat bread, plus carrots and celery with hummus.
- Dinner: Curry chicken, brown rice, lentils.

You can drink a glass of wine with each dinner to satisfy the MIND diet recommendations. Nuts can also make a great snack. Most salad dressings you find at the store are not made primarily with olive oil, but you can easily make your own salad dressing at home. To make a simple balsamic vinaigrette, combine three parts extra virgin olive oil with one-part balsamic vinegar. Add a little Dijon mustard, salt and pepper, then mix well.

When looking at MIND diet meals, it is good to form a MIND diet meal plan. Some of the top recipes for the MIND diet include:

Breakfast:

- Six ounces of Greek yogurt
- ½ cup of blueberries
- ½ cup of strawberries

Lunch: A salad with-

- 1 cup of romaine lettuce
- 1 cup of fresh cucumber slices
- ½ cup of tomato wedges
- 1 tsp of low-calorie Italian dressing
- 1 tbsp of sunflower seeds

Dinner:

- 3 ounces of salmon
- 1 tsp tarragon

- 1 tsp mustard

- ½ cup couscous

- ½ cup zucchini

- 4 asparagus spears

- 1 cup lima beans

- 5 ounces of red wine

Snack:

- ½ cup assorted nuts (almonds, pecans, cashews, walnuts)

Snack:

- 1 cup of hummus

- Assorted carrot sticks or celery sticks

These recipes could form the foundation of a MIND diet shopping list, helping you find the right MIND diet foods.

The Guidelines for the MIND Diet – The MIND Diet Pyramid

In some cases, it might be easier for people to look at the MIND diet in the form of a diet pyramid. As with any pyramid, it is essential to start at the bottom and work out. Therefore, let's begin by looking at the two diets that form the foundation of the MIND diet. The first component is called a Mediterranean or Medi diet. The Medi diet is named in this manner because it is a traditional diet of people who live in the Mediterranean area of the world. Several foods commonly appear in the diet. The goal is to stick to plant food and minimally-processed foods. Some of the most popular foods include cereal grains, legumes, fruits, nuts, vegetables. Also, fish is the primary source of protein in the Medi diet. Fish has already been found to be helpful to the neurological system. Even though small amounts of meat, dairy, and alcohol are scattered throughout the Medi diet, these are relatively small components. The other central pillar of the MIND diet is the DASH diet. This diet was initially designed to help people who struggle with cardiovascular issues by providing heart-healthy foods. The acronym stands for the Dietary Plan to Stop Hypertension. Given that elevated blood pressure can increase the risk of neurological problems, it makes sense that this diet would be included in the MIND diet. The goal of the diet is to emphasize fruits, low-fat dairy products, and vegetables. In addition, this diet includes whole grains, fish, nuts, and poultry.

Finally, this diet also reduces red meat, fats, sweets, and beverages containing a high amount of sugar.

In this manner, the DASH diet and the Medi diet form the pyramid's foundation that makes up the MIND diet. Overall, the MIND diet emphasizes natural, plant-based foods and increases the consumption of berries, green leafy vegetables, and fish while limiting foods with saturated fats. Now, turning the MIND diet into a pyramid, it is time to work from the ground-up. Those following recipes for the MIND diet should:

- Eat at least one dark green salad and one additional vegetable every day.
- Eat at least a single serving of nuts every day.
- Eat beans or other legumes every other day.
- Eat berries at least twice per week.
- Eat poultry at least twice per week.
- Eat fish at least once per week.

Finally, at the top of the pyramid, a single glass of wine every day, as long as a physician has approved this.

Of course, there are many people interested in pursuing the MIND diet but are a bit worried about how much the MIND diet is going to cost. There is a false perception that eating healthy is expensive. The good news is that this is not the case.

By taking a closer look at the most popular foods on the MIND diet, it is easy to see that the diet is relatively inexpensive. Vegetables and dark leafy greens are not expensive. Compared to other types of meat (particularly red meat), poultry is significantly less costly. Even though seafood and olive oil can be expensive, individuals on the MIND diet do not have to use a lot of olive oil and seafood is only required once per week. Therefore, the MIND diet does not have to be expensive.

Overall, this diet seeks to reduce the decline in brain health that has been associated with dementia and Alzheimer's disease. Even though this diet is still relatively new, there is a lot of evidence that shows that it can help people preserve their mental faculties by reducing the risk of dementia. In particular, those with a family history of neurological problems may want to consider starting this diet of brain-friendly foods at a younger age.

How Easy is the MIND Diet to Follow?

There is a saying that a diet is only helpful if it can be followed. Therefore, is the MIND diet easy to follow? Recently, a US News and World Report article listed the "Best Diets" and the MIND diet was included seven times. The MIND diet was ranked in the top five for five separate categories (including healthy eating) and also took the best slot as the easiest diet to follow. While diets do require some discipline, the MIND diet is one of the easiest to follow.

How Much Should You Exercise on the MIND Diet?

One of the most critical tactics for improving overall health is a healthy diet and exercise. While there are no specific studies on the MIND diet and exercise, activity can still impact brain health.

Health Benefits of the MIND Diet

Brain Health

In numerous human and animal studies, foods highlighted in the MIND diet reduced the incidence of Alzheimer's and dementia, and improved memory. This was particularly so in those with healthy brain function or at the very early stages of cognitive decline.

Alzheimer's and Dementia

In a clinical trial of 923 people, modest compliance to the MIND diet for 4.5 years decreased the incidence of Alzheimer's disease by 53% in those over 60 years of age. In comparison, people had to comply very strictly to the Mediterranean or DASH diet to see similar results.

The main foods that protect against dementia and Alzheimer's disease are precisely those highlighted in MIND diet (extra virgin olive oil, whole grains, nuts and legumes, and reduced dairy), according to comprehensive reviews on nutrition and brain health. In observational studies of between 2,000 and 10,000 people aged 55 years or older, eating MIND diet foods protected against Alzheimer's and dementia. On the other hand, eating white bread, high-fat dairy products, eggs, meat, fried foods, and sweets was linked to an increased rate of disease. Fish high in omega-3 fatty acids and vitamin D (salmon, herring, mackerel, sardines) should be prioritized. Omega-3s from fish and marine oils were linked to prevention and improvement of Alzheimer's disease. The MIND diet limits alcohol consumption to 1 drink per day, a quantity that protected against Alzheimer's and dementia in observational studies. Inversely, both abstinence and heavier consumption (more than 2 drinks per day) were linked with greater incidence of disease

Memory and Cognition

In a clinical trial of about 500 older people (>70 years of age), the Mediterranean diet enhanced with olive oil or nuts improved cognition more than a low-fat diet. Specifically, polyphenols in olive oil improve learning and memory, according to reviews of human and animal studies. Eating MIND-diet foods improved cognitive function including memory, attention and visual-spatial skills in observational studies of over 23,000 people (aged

58 years or more). Lower intake of vegetables and legumes, specifically, was linked to cognitive decline. Each of the specific foods highlighted in the MIND diet (extra virgin olive oil, berries, leafy green vegetables) improved cognition, learning, memory, and reduced age-related brain dysfunction and oxidative damage in rats and mice.

Inflammation

Chronic inflammation can trigger or worsen many diseases, including Alzheimer's, heart and autoimmune diseases. In some cases, eating mostly MIND-diet-friendly nutrient-dense, plant-based foods and eliminating high-fat and sugary foods can reduce inflammation. Eating MIND diet foods (legumes, whole grains, vegetables, olive oil) for at least 12 weeks lowered markers of inflammation (analysis of 17 clinical trials and about 2,300 people). In a clinical trial with 164 people at high risk for heart disease, a Mediterranean diet that included 1.5 oz of extra virgin olive oil and ¼ cup of nuts per day reduced inflammatory markers by up to 95%

compared to low-fat diets in older people (55 – 80 years of age)

Olive oil is the key anti-inflammatory ingredient of the MIND diet. The evidence to back up its benefits is abundant. For example, olive oil reduced inflammation in people over 50 years of age, having a stronger effect in those at higher risk for heart disease (reviews of clinical studies of about 500 people and observational studies of over 40,000 people). Consuming extra virgin olive oil has also been linked to reduced inflammation in autoimmune diseases like rheumatoid arthritis, IBS, amyotrophic lateral sclerosis (ALS), and multiple sclerosis (observational and clinical reviews). Polyphenols from olive oil and red wine reduced inflammation in human cells. Antioxidant polyphenols are possibly the main anti-inflammatory substances in these foods

The MIND diet recommends eating plant-based foods high in fiber, complex carbs, vitamins, minerals, healthy fats, and phytochemicals. MIND diet foods reduced the rate of heart disease, deaths from heart disease, total cholesterol, and HDL cholesterol compared to lower-fat diets, according to meta-analyses of observational and clinical trials. Extra virgin olive oil, the primary fat in the MIND diet, helped prevent heart failure, plaque build-up in the arteries, irregular heartbeat and heart disease (review of clinical and observational studies). Flavonoids, abundant in berries, were linked to lower LDL cholesterol, triglycerides, lower blood pressure, as well as improved heart health overall (clinical, observational, and animal studies).

Diabetes

Eating high amounts of whole grains, fruits and vegetables improved blood sugar control and reduced overall incidence of Type 2 diabetes by about 20% compared to low-fat diets (review of meta-analyses and 5 clinical trials). One analysis of over 400 observational studies explored the relationship between major food groups in the MIND diet (whole grains, vegetables, nuts, legumes, and fish) and type 2 diabetes. They found that:

- Decreasing the consumption of "high risk" foods (red and processed meats, sugary drinks) reduced the incidence of type 2 diabetes threefold;
- Eating optimal amounts of whole grains (2 servings/day), fruits (2-3 servings/day), and vegetables (2-3 servings/day) reduced the incidence of type 2 diabetes by 42%
- Eating 50g/day of whole grains alone reduced the incidence of type 2 diabetes by 25%

Weight Loss

The MIND diet is designed for brain health, but the focus on whole, plant-based foods and the reduction of sweets, dairy, fried and fast foods may promote healthy weight loss. The diet is also rich in fiber and low in high-calorie foods. Plant-based foods (legumes and whole grains) prevented weight gain and obesity better than high-protein, low-fat, and low-glycemic-index diets in observational and clinical studies. Metabolic syndrome is a cluster of conditions that increase the risk of obesity. Eating olive oil, vegetables, whole grains, legumes, and nuts decreased the rate of metabolic syndrome by 35%

and reduced the likelihood of weight gain in an observational study of almost 800 young adults.

Depression

MIND-like diets, high in plant-based foods, reduced the rate of depression in several studies (clinical and observational). The protective effects are likely from eating a combination of these foods, as opposed to taking isolated nutrients. In a clinical trial of 95 postmenopausal women, the DASH diet (one of the parent diets of the MIND diet) for 14 weeks, improved mood and reduced symptoms of depression. In an observational study of almost 16,000 adults, sticking to the Mediterranean diet for 10 years was linked with a decreased incidence of depression. These results were attributed to foods also found in the MIND diet (vegetables, legumes, whole grains, nuts, fish).

Parkinson's Disease

In observational studies of over 1.5 million people, diets rich in foods common to the Mediterranean and MIND diets reduced the incidence of Parkinson's disease by 13%.

In another observational study of over 700 people older people, the MIND diet slowed the progression of Parkinson's disease symptoms such as tremors and poor balance.

Longevity

In observational studies of over 3,000 people, a MIND-like diet was linked to a longer lifespan in people over 65 years of age. This effect was associated with a slower rate at which the telomeres get shortened, a key indicator of biological aging

Cancer Research

Heavy consumption of MIND diet foods (especially vegetables, legumes, olive oil, and whole grains) was associated with reduced rates of cancer. It also reduced the number of deaths from various cancers, including colon, breast, stomach, pancreas, prostate, liver, and head and neck cancers (reviews of clinical and observational studies). Phytochemicals and antioxidants in berries and olive oil prevented colon cancer or and delayed its spreading in numerous studies (observational, clinical, animal, and cellular). Consuming nuts more than 8 times/month for over 4 years was linked to a reduced rate of cancer and death in over 19,000 people. This study suggests that MIND diet recommendations of nut intake on the higher ranger (5 servings per week) may also protect against cancer

The current research on the MIND diet has not been able to show exactly how it works. However, the scientists who created the diet think it may work by reducing oxidative stress and inflammation. Oxidative stress occurs when unstable molecules called free radicals accumulate in the body in large quantities. This often causes damage to cells. The brain is especially vulnerable to this type of damage. Inflammation is your body's natural response to injury and infection. But if it's not properly regulated, inflammation can also be harmful and contribute to many chronic diseases. Together, oxidative stress and inflammation can be quite detrimental to the brain. In recent years, they've been the focus of some interventions to prevent and treat Alzheimer's disease. Following the Mediterranean and DASH diets has been associated with lower levels of oxidative stress and inflammation. Because the MIND diet is a hybrid of these two diets, the foods that make up the MIND diet probably also have antioxidant and anti-inflammatory effects. The antioxidants in berries and the vitamin E in olive oil, green leafy vegetables and nuts are thought to benefit brain function by protecting the brain from oxidative stress. Additionally, the omega-3 fatty acids found in fatty fish are well-known for their ability to lower inflammation in the brain, and have been associated with slower loss of brain function.

The MIND Diet May Reduce Harmful Beta-Amyloid Proteins
Researchers also believe the MIND diet may benefit the brain by reducing potentially harmful beta-amyloid proteins. Beta-amyloid proteins are protein fragments found naturally in the body. However, they can accumulate and form plaques that build up in the brain, disrupting communication between brain cells and eventually leading to brain cell death. In fact, many scientists believe these plaques are one of the primary causes of Alzheimer's disease. Animal and test-tube studies suggest that the antioxidants and vitamins that

many MIND diet foods contain may help prevent the formation of beta-amyloid plaques in the brain. Additionally, the MIND diet limits foods that contain saturated fats and trans fats, which studies have shown can increase beta-amyloid protein levels in mice's brains. Human observational studies have found that consuming these fats was associated with a doubled risk of Alzheimer's disease. However, it is important to note that this type of research is not able to determine cause and effect. Higher-quality, controlled studies are needed to discover exactly how the MIND diet may benefit brain health.

- The primary purpose of the MIND dict is to boost the performance of the brain in old age. It also offers several benefits other than regulating the brain's functionality.

- It provides a complete range of nutrition according to a person's age.

- Additionally, its health benefits are easy to observe, unlike strict diet plans.

- MIND diet is useful for reducing the risk of dementia, which generally occurs in old age and can be life-threatening.

- Even people who are not at risk of developing neurodegenerative diseases like Parkinson's or Alzheimer's disease can follow this diet.

- This diet is useful for healthy weight loss and maintaining BMI.

- The MIND diet provides many antioxidants which are required for the body's internal functioning.

- This diet balances the cholesterol levels and consequently reduces chronic conditions like heart diseases.

- One major benefit of the MIND diet is th

- at it will make a person feel and stay younger.

Watermelon Fruit Bowl

Recipe Summary

All of your favorite fruits, lightly sweetened, served in a watermelon 'bowl'.

Prep:30 mins

Cook:5 mins

Additional:15 mins

Total:50 mins

Servings:20

Yield:20 servings

Ingredients

1 large watermelon

1 cantaloupe, halved and seeded

1 honeydew melon, halved and seeded

2 (15 ounce) cans mandarin oranges, drained

2 (20 ounce) cans pineapple chunks, drained

2 cups halved fresh strawberries

2 cups seedless grapes

½ cup water

¼ cup white sugar

2 tablespoons grated lemon zest

Directions

Step 1

With a large, sharp knife, remove the top 1/4 section of the watermelon. With a melon baller, scoop flesh from inside of watermelon, removing as many seeds as possible. Leave 1/2 inch of flesh inside the shell of the watermelon. Scoop cantaloupe and honeydew in the same manner, removing as much flesh as possible, and discarding the rinds. Refrigerate fruits separately until ready to assemble.

Step 2

In a small saucepan over medium-high heat, bring water and sugar to a boil. Remove from heat, and continue stirring until sugar has completely dissolved. Add lemon zest, and set aside to cool

Step 3

To serve, place watermelon balls, cantaloupe, honeydew, oranges, pineapple, strawberries, and grapes, in a large mixing bowl. Pour syrup over, and toss thoroughly. Transfer mixture to watermelon bowl, and serve. Set aside any fruit mixture that will not fit. There will be enough fruit to refill the bowl.

Nutrition Facts

Per Serving: 179 calories; protein 2.8g; carbohydrates 45.4g; fat 0.7g; sodium 23.4mg.

Pears and Dried Fruits in a Tagine
Recipe Summary

Pears and other dried fruits with lemon and honey cooked in a tagine.

Prep:10 mins

Cook:40 mins

Additional:10 mins

Total:1 hr

Servings:4

Yield:4 servings

Ingredients

1 organic lemon

2 tablespoons honey

1 (3 inch) cinnamon stick

1 vanilla bean, cut in half lengthwise

2 pears - peeled, cored, and quartered

8 pitted prunes

8 dried apricots

¼ cup blanched whole almonds

⅛ cup pine nuts

Directions

Step 1

Preheat the oven to 375 degrees F (190 degrees C).

Step 2

Wash lemon and remove peel with a knife, trying to keep it in one long string. Squeeze juice from 1/2 of the lemon into a small saucepan. Add honey, cinnamon stick, and vanilla bean. Bring to a boil, then lower heat and simmer until fragrant and syrupy, about 5 minutes

Step 3

Arrange pears, core-sides up, in a tagine. Add prunes, apricots, almonds, and lemon peel around the pears and on top if necessary. Pour lemon juice mixture over top allowing cinnamon stick and vanilla bean halves to fall into the tagine. Cover

Step 4

Cook in the preheated oven for 20 minutes. Remove from the oven and take off the cover, allowing any condensation to fall back into the tagine. Turn pears over and add pine nuts. Replace the cover and cook for 10 minutes. Turn the oven off, and allow the tagine to sit in the hot oven until sauce thickens a bit, about 10 minutes. Serve.

Cook's Note:

You can use agave in place of honey

Nutrition Facts

Per Serving: 266 calories; protein 4.7g; carbohydrates 54.2g; fat 7g; sodium 5.1mg.

Juicy Slow Cooker Chicken Breast for Any Diet

Recipe Summary

Prep: 10 mins

Cook: 6 hrs

Total: 6 hrs 10 mins

Servings: 4

Yield: 4 servings

Ingredients

- 1 pound skinless, boneless chicken breast halves
- 1 (14.5 ounce) can petite diced tomatoes
- ¼ onion, chopped (Optional)
- 1 teaspoon Italian seasoning (Optional)
- 1 clove garlic, minced (Optional)

Directions

Step 1

Arrange chicken in a slow cooker. Pour tomatoes over chicken; add onion, Italian seasoning, and garlic.

Step 2

Cook on Low for 6 to 8 hours.

Cook's Note:

You can use any type of herb in place of the Italian seasoning.

Nutrition Facts

Per Serving: 144 calories; protein 23.1g; carbohydrates 5.2g; fat 2.4g; cholesterol 58.5mg; sodium 208mg.

Balsamic Marinated Chicken Breasts

Recipe Summary

Prep: 15 mins

Cook: 40 mins

Additional: 30 mins

Total: 1 hr 25 mins

Servings: 4

Yield: 4 chicken breasts

Ingredients

- ¾ cup balsamic vinegar
- ½ cup water
- 1 teaspoon dried minced onion
- ½ teaspoon crushed red pepper flakes
- ½ teaspoon dried minced garlic
- ¼ teaspoon salt
- ¼ teaspoon ground black pepper
- ¼ teaspoon paprika
- ¼ teaspoon crushed dried rosemary

- ¼ teaspoon dried parsley flakes

- ¼ teaspoon chili powder

- ⅛ teaspoon dried oregano

- 4 (6 ounce) skinless, boneless chicken breast halves

Directions

Step 1

Whisk together the balsamic vinegar, water, onion, red pepper flakes, garlic, salt, pepper, paprika, rosemary, parsley, chili powder, and oregano in a bowl, and pour into a resealable plastic bag. Add the chicken breasts, coat with the marinade, squeeze out excess air, and seal the bag. Marinate in the refrigerator 30 minutes to overnight.

Step 2

Preheat oven to 400 degrees F (200 degrees C). Line a baking sheet with aluminum foil, or lightly grease a broiler pan. Remove the chicken breasts from the marinade, and shake off excess. Discard the remaining marinade, and place the chicken breasts onto the baking sheet.

Step 3

Bake in the preheated oven until the chicken breasts are golden brown and no longer pink in the center, 30 to 40 minutes. An instant-read thermometer inserted into the center should reach 165 degrees F (74 degrees C).

Nutrition Facts

Per Serving: 222 calories; protein 35.7g; carbohydrates 8g; fat 4.3g; cholesterol 96.9mg; sodium 244.3mg.

Lemon Garlic Chicken Breasts

Recipe Summary

Prep: 10 mins

Cook: 25 mins

Total: 35 mins

Servings: 4

Yield: 4 servings

Ingredients

- cooking spray

- 1 clove garlic, minced

- 4 skinless, boneless chicken breast halves

- salt and ground black pepper to taste

- ¾ cup chicken broth

- 1 tablespoon lemon juice

Directions

Step 1

Lightly spray a nonstick skillet with cooking spray and place over low heat; cook and stir garlic until fragrant and lightly browned, 2 to 3 minutes.

Step 2

Season chicken with salt and pepper and place in skillet with garlic; cook over medium heat until browned on both sides, 10 to 12 minutes. Add chicken broth and lemon juice; bring to a boil. Reduce heat to medium-low, cover skillet, and simmer until chicken is no longer pink in the center, 10 to 15 minutes. An instant-read thermometer inserted into the center should read at least 165 degrees F (74 degrees C).

Step 3

Transfer chicken to a serving dish, reserving liquid in skillet. Continue simmering liquid until slightly reduced, about 3 minutes. Pour liquid over chicken.

Nutrition Facts

Per Serving: 131 calories; protein 23.8g; carbohydrates 0.8g; fat 2.9g; cholesterol 65.5mg; sodium 275.2mg.

Alabama White BBQ Sauce

Recipe Summary

Prep: 5 mins

Total: 5 mins

Servings: 12

Yield: 1 1/2 cups

Ingredients

- 1 cup mayonnaise

- ⅓ cup apple cider vinegar

- 3 teaspoons water

- 1 teaspoon Worcestershire sauce

- ½ teaspoon kosher salt

- ½ teaspoon garlic powder

- ½ teaspoon onion powder

- ½ teaspoon freshly ground black pepper

- ¼ teaspoon hot sauce

Directions

Step 1

Combine mayonnaise, vinegar, water, Worcestershire sauce, salt, garlic powder, onion powder, pepper, and hot sauce in a bowl; mix until thoroughly combined.

Nutrition Facts

Per Serving: 134 calories; protein 0.2g; carbohydrates 0.9g; fat 14.6g; cholesterol 7mg; sodium 191.8mg.

Recipe Summary

Prep: 15 mins

Total: 15 mins

Servings: 64

Yield: 4 pints

Ingredients

- 1 (17 ounce) jar Major Grey chutney
- 4 ½ ounces pickled walnuts (Optional)
- 1 (14 ounce) bottle ketchup
- 1 (10 fluid ounce) bottle steak sauce
- 1 (10 fluid ounce) bottle Worcestershire sauce
- 1 (12 ounce) bottle tomato-based chili sauce
- 1 dash hot pepper sauce (such as Tabasco®), or to taste

Directions

 Step 1

Mix chutney, pickled walnuts, ketchup, steak sauce, Worcestershire sauce, chili sauce, and hot pepper sauce in a large bowl. Refrigerate until ready to use. Serve at room temperature.

Cook's Note:

Pickled walnuts are optional. Obtainable at specialty gourmet shops.

Nutrition Facts

Per Serving: 27 calories; protein 0.3g; carbohydrates 6.7g; fat 0.1g; sodium 184.3mg.

Comeback Sauce
Recipe Summary

Prep: 5 mins

Additional: 2 hrs

Total: 2 hrs 5 mins

Servings: 10

Yield: 1 1/4 cups

Ingredients

- ¾ cup mayonnaise
- ¼ cup ketchup
- ¼ cup chili sauce
- 1 tablespoon fresh lemon juice
- 1 teaspoon Worcestershire sauce
- ½ teaspoon dry mustard powder
- ½ teaspoon onion powder
- ½ teaspoon hot pepper sauce
- ¼ teaspoon garlic powder
- ¼ teaspoon paprika

Directions

Step 1

Combine mayonnaise, ketchup, chili sauce, lemon juice, Worcestershire sauce, dry mustard, onion powder, hot sauce, garlic powder, and paprika in a small bowl; whisk until well combined.

Step 2

Refrigerate for at least 2 hours to allow the flavors to meld, though overnight is even better.

Nutrition Facts

Per Serving: 134 calories; protein 0.5g; carbohydrates 4.2g; fat 13.2g; cholesterol 6.3mg; sodium 259mg.

Tequila-Lime Chicken

Recipe Summary

Prep: 10 mins

Cook: 35 mins

Additional: 1 hr

Total: 1 hr 45 mins

Servings: 4

Yield: 4 servings

Ingredients

- 3 skinless, boneless chicken breasts
- ½ cup tequila

- 1 lime, zested and juiced
- ¼ teaspoon garlic powder, divided
- ¼ teaspoon chili powder, divided
- 3 ounces shredded Mexican-style cheese blend

Directions

Step 1

Arrange chicken breasts in a baking dish; add tequila and juice of 1/2 a lime. Sprinkle 1/2 of the lime zest, 1/2 of the garlic powder, and 1/2 of the chili powder over the chicken. Cover dish with plastic wrap and marinate in the refrigerator for 30 minutes.

Step 2

Turn chicken breasts; sprinkle remaining lime juice, lime zest, garlic powder, and chili powder on top. Cover again and marinate in the refrigerator for another 30 minutes.

Step 3

Preheat the oven to 425 degrees F (220 degrees C). Uncover baking dish and discard tequila-lime marinade.

Step 4

Bake chicken in the preheated oven for 25 minutes. Sprinkle Mexican-style cheese over the chicken and continue to bake until the chicken is no longer pink in the center and the juices run clear, about 10 minutes more. An instant-read thermometer inserted into the center should read at least 165 degrees F (74 degrees C).

Editor's Note:

Nutrition data for this recipe includes the full amount of marinade ingredients. The actual amount of marinade consumed will vary.

Nutrition Facts

Per Serving: 244 calories; protein 22.5g; carbohydrates 1.7g; fat 8.8g; cholesterol 68.8mg; sodium 207mg.

Beets with Onion and Cumin
Recipe Summary

Prep: 15 mins

Cook: 45 mins

Total: 1 hr

Servings: 4

Yield: 4 servings

Ingredients

- 2 tablespoons canola oil
- 1 small onion, chopped
- 1 clove garlic, minced
- 1 ½ teaspoons cumin seed
- 2 tablespoons all-purpose flour
- 5 medium beets, peeled and quartered
- 2 tomatoes - peeled, seeded and chopped
- 1 ½ cups water
- 1 teaspoon salt

Directions

Step 1

Heat a medium saucepan over medium-high heat. Pour in oil and saute onion and garlic until translucent. Mix in cumin seed and saute an additional 2 minutes. Sprinkle in flour and saute 1 minute more.

Step 2

Stir in beets, tomatoes, water, and salt. Reduce heat to low, cover pan with lid, and allow to simmer 30 to 45 minutes, until beets are tender.

Nutrition Facts

Per Serving: 139 calories; protein 2.9g; carbohydrates 16.7g; fat 7.5g; sodium 849.3mg.

Greek Green Beans

Recipe Summary

Prep: 20 mins

Cook: 55 mins

Total: 1 hr 15 mins

Servings: 8

Yield: 8 servings

Ingredients

- ¾ cup olive oil
- 2 cups chopped onions
- 1 clove garlic, minced
- 2 pounds fresh green beans, rinsed and trimmed
- 3 large tomatoes, diced
- 2 teaspoons sugar
- salt to taste

Directions

Step 1

Heat the olive oil in a large skillet over medium heat. Cook and stir the onions and garlic in the skillet until tender.

Step 2

Mix the green beans, tomatoes, sugar, and salt into the skillet. Reduce heat to low, and continue cooking 45 minutes, or until beans are soft.

Nutrition Facts

Per Serving: 243 calories; protein 3g; carbohydrates 14.6g; fat 20.6g; sodium 11.8mg.

Summerly Squash

Recipe Summary

Prep: 15 mins

Cook: 30 mins

Total: 45 mins

Servings: 6

Yield: 6 servings

Ingredients

- 2 tablespoons vegetable oil
- 1 small onion, sliced
- 2 medium tomatoes, coarsely chopped
- 1 teaspoon salt
- ¼ teaspoon pepper
- 2 small zucchini, cut into 1/2 inch slices

- 2 small yellow summer squash, cut into 1/2-inch slices
- 1 bay leaf
- ½ teaspoon dried basil

Directions

Step 1

Heat the oil in a large skillet over medium heat. Cook and stir the onion about 5 minutes, until tender. Mix in the tomatoes, and season with salt and pepper. Continue to cook and stir about 5 minutes. Mix in the zucchini, yellow squash, bay leaf, and basil. Cover, reduce heat to low, and simmer 20 minutes, stirring occasionally. Remove bay leaf before serving.

Nutrition Facts

Per Serving: 65 calories; protein 1.5g; carbohydrates 5.4g; fat 4.8g; sodium 394.9mg.

Vegetable Medley II
Recipe Summary

Prep: 20 mins

Cook: 15 mins

Total: 35 mins

Servings: 4

Yield: 4 servings

Ingredients

- cooking spray
- 1 tomato, diced
- 1 pinch garlic pepper seasoning
- 2 cups fresh mushrooms, sliced
- 2 yellow squash, cubed
- 2 zucchini, cubed

Directions

Step 1

Spray a large skillet with cooking spray and add tomatoes. Cook over medium heat for 5 minutes and add garlic pepper. Stir in mushrooms, squash, and zucchini. Simmer until vegetables are tender-crisp, 10 to 15 minutes.

Nutrition Facts

Per Serving: 66 calories; protein 3.3g; carbohydrates 12.6g; fat 1.5g; sodium 201.7mg.

Broccoli, Leek, and Potato Soup

Recipe Summary

Prep: 20 mins

Cook: 40 mins

Total: 1 hr

Servings: 6

Yield: 6 servings

Ingredients

- 4 slices bacon, diced
- 2 tablespoons olive oil
- 2 tablespoons butter
- 3 large leeks, chopped
- 1 onion, chopped
- 3 stalks celery, chopped
- 3 cups chicken stock

- 3 Yukon Gold potatoes, cubed

- 1 teaspoon herbes de Provence

- ½ teaspoon ground coriander

- ½ teaspoon fennel seed, crushed

- ½ teaspoon salt

- 1 teaspoon ground black pepper

- 3 cups broccoli florets

- 2 ½ cups whole milk

- 3 green onions, chopped (Optional)

Directions

Step 1

Stir the bacon and olive oil in a large pot over medium heat until the bacon has turned golden brown and released its grease, about 7 minutes. Add the butter, leeks, onion, and celery. Cook and stir until the leeks have softened, about 7 minutes.

Step 2

Pour in the chicken stock, potatoes, herbes de Provence, coriander, fennel, salt, and pepper. Bring to a boil over high heat, then reduce heat to medium-low, cover, and simmer until the potatoes are just beginning to turn tender, about 8 minutes. Stir in the broccoli, and simmer 5 minutes. Add the milk, and continue simmering until the vegetables are tender, about 5 minutes more.

Step 3

Pour the soup into a blender, filling the pitcher no more than halfway full. Hold down the lid of the blender with a folded kitchen towel, and carefully start the blender, using a few quick pulses to get the soup moving before leaving it on to puree. Puree in batches until smooth and pour into a clean pot. Alternately, you can use a stick blender and puree the soup right in the cooking pot. Season to taste with additional salt and pepper; sprinkle with chopped green onions to serve.

Nutrition Facts

Per Serving: 297 calories; protein 10g; carbohydrates 33g; fat 15g; cholesterol 27.3mg; sodium 794.7mg.

Chocolate-y Iced Mocha
Recipe Summary

Prep: 5 mins

Cook: 1 min

Total: 6 mins

Servings: 1

Yield: 1 serving

Ingredients

- 1 ¼ cups cold coffee, divided
- 1 envelope low-calorie hot cocoa mix
- ice cubes, or as needed
- ½ cup unsweetened almond milk
- 2 tablespoons sugar-free chocolate syrup, or more to taste

Directions

Step 1

Heat 1/4 cup coffee in microwave in a mug until warmed, about 30 seconds. Stir cocoa mix into the coffee until dissolved.

Step 2

Fill a large glass with ice cubes. Pour 1 cup cold coffee and almond milk over the ice cubes; stir the cocoa mixture and chocolate syrup into the coffee and almond milk.

Nutrition Facts

Per Serving: 105 calories; protein 5.2g; carbohydrates 16.7g; fat 1.8g; cholesterol 2.9mg; sodium 255.3mg.

Sugar-Free Cream Cheese Frosting
Recipe Summary

Prep: 5 mins

Total: 5 mins

Servings: 12

Yield: 12 servings

Ingredients

- 1 (8 ounce) package reduced-fat cream cheese, softened
- ½ cup granular sucrolose sweetener, or more to taste

- 1 (8 ounce) container frozen whipped topping, thawed
- 1 teaspoon vanilla extract

Directions

Step 1

Beat cream cheese and sucralose sweetener together in a bowl using an electric mixer until smooth and creamy; stir in whipped topping and vanilla extract until smooth.

Nutrition Facts

Per Serving: 104 calories; protein 2.2g; carbohydrates 5.7g; fat 8.1g; cholesterol 10.6mg; sodium 60.7mg.

Apricot/Cranberry Chutney

Recipe Summary

Prep: 10 mins

Cook: 15 mins

Additional: 5 mins

Total: 30 mins

Servings: 12

Yield: 12 servings

Ingredients

- ¼ cup diced dried apricots
- 1 (12 ounce) package fresh cranberries
- ½ cup raisins
- ¾ teaspoon ground cinnamon
- ¼ teaspoon ground ginger
- ¼ teaspoon ground allspice
- 1 pinch ground cloves
- 1 cup water
- ¾ cup white sugar
- ½ cup cider vinegar

Directions

Step 1

In a medium bowl, mix together the apricots, cranberries, raisins, cinnamon, ginger, allspice, and cloves.

Step 2

In a medium saucepan, boil water and sugar, stirring constantly, until sugar is dissolved. Add the dried fruit mixture and vinegar. Bring to a boil, reduce heat, and simmer for 10 minutes. Remove from heat, and allow to cool for 5 minutes. Serve immediately, or refrigerate in a covered container.

Nutrition Facts

Per Serving: 89 calories; protein 0.4g; carbohydrates 22.7g; fat 0.1g; sodium 2.3mg.

Keto-Friendly Bread
Recipe Summary

Prep: 15 mins

Cook: 35 mins

Additional: 10 mins

Total: 1 hr

Servings: 8

Yield: 8 servings

Ingredients

- cooking spray
- 6 eggs, separated
- ¼ teaspoon cream of tartar
- 6 tablespoons coconut flour
- 6 tablespoons almond flour
- 2 tablespoons arrowroot powder
- 1 teaspoon gluten-free baking powder
- ½ teaspoon kosher salt
- ¼ cup coconut oil, melted and cooled
- 1 tablespoon honey

Directions

Step 1

Preheat the oven to 350 degrees F (175 degrees C). Spray a 4x8-inch loaf pan with cooking spray.

Step 2

Beat egg whites in a glass, metal, or ceramic bowl until foamy. Gradually add cream of tartar, continuing to beat until soft peaks form. Set aside.

Step 3

Combine coconut flour, almond flour, arrowroot powder, baking powder, and salt in a bowl and mix well.

Step 4

Beat egg yolks using an electric mixer in a bowl until thick. Add coconut oil and honey; mix well. Add flour mixture and stir until well combined. Fold in 1/4 of the beaten egg whites until incorporated. Add 1/2 the remaining egg whites and gently fold until only small amounts of egg whites are visible. Repeat with remaining egg whites. Pour mixture into prepared loaf pan and smooth the top.

Step 5

Bake in the preheated oven until nicely golden brown on top, about 35 minutes. Remove from oven, set on a wire rack, and let cool for 10 minutes. Run a knife around the sides, tip out bread onto a rack, and let cool completely.

Cook's Note:

The bread can be flavored in any way you like, for example, with a little artificial sweetener and almond, orange, or lemon extract for a breakfast or dessert treat, or herbs for a savory side.

Nutrition Facts

Per Serving: 181 calories; protein 6.3g; carbohydrates 9.8g; fat 13.7g; cholesterol 122.8mg; sodium 227.3mg.

Rickyrootbeer
Recipe Summary

Prep: 5 mins

Total: 5 mins

Servings: 1

Yield: 1 drink

Ingredients

- ½ fluid ounce vanilla vodka
- ½ fluid ounce Irish cream liqueur
- 4 fluid ounces root beer

Directions

Step 1

Pour the vodka and Irish cream into a shot glass. Pour the root beer into a tumbler. Drop the entire shot glass into the root beer and drink immediately.

Nutrition Facts

Per Serving: 140 calories; protein 0g; carbohydrates 19.9g; fat 0g; cholesterol 0mg; sodium 17.2mg.

Diet Soup

Recipe Summary

Prep: 20 mins

Cook: 30 mins

Total: 50 mins

Servings: 8

Yield: 8 servings

Ingredients

- 1 medium head cabbage, chopped
- 1 onion, chopped
- 3 large carrots, chopped
- 3 stalks celery, chopped
- 3 tomatoes, chopped
- 16 ounces frozen green beans
- 2 (1 ounce) packages dry onion soup mix
- 6 cups water

Directions

Step 1

Combine water, soup mix, and vegetables in a large stock pot. Bring to a boil. Reduce heat, and simmer until the vegetables are tender.

Nutrition Facts

Per Serving: 94 calories; protein 3.6g; carbohydrates 21g; fat 0.5g; sodium 672.9mg.

Turkey Frame Vegetable Soup

Recipe Summary

Prep: 1 hr 30 mins

Cook: 1 hr 20 mins

Additional: 8 hrs

Total: 10 hrs 50 mins

Servings: 8

Yield: 8 servings

Ingredients

- 1 turkey carcass
- 2 carrots, chopped
- 2 stalks celery, cut into 2 inch pieces
- 1 onions, chopped
- 4 cloves garlic, minced
- 4 sprigs fresh parsley
- 12 black peppercorns
- 2 bay leaves
- 1 teaspoon dried thyme
- 1 tablespoon chicken bouillon granules
- 8 cups water

- water to cover
- 1 turnip, peeled and cubed
- 2 parsnips, peeled and sliced
- 3 carrots, chopped
- ½ cup frozen green beans
- ½ cup frozen green peas
- 1 (15 ounce) can red beans, drained and rinsed
- ¼ cup chopped fresh parsley

Directions

Step 1

Place turkey carcass in a large pot over high heat. Add the carrots, celery, onion, garlic, parsley sprigs, peppercorns, bay leaves, thyme, chicken bouillon granules, water and enough water to cover all. Bring to a boil, uncovered, then reduce heat to medium low and let simmer for 1 1/2 hours.

Step 2

Remove the turkey carcass and allow it to cool. Remove any meat from the carcass, cut into bite-sized pieces and set aside. Strain the stock through a sieve OR a colander covered with cheesecloth into another large pot. Discard the unstrained ingredients. Place the turkey meat into the pot, cover and refrigerate overnight.

Step 3

The next day, use a slotted spoon to remove the fat that has solidified on top of the stock. Return the stock to a large pot over high heat, add the turnip, parsnips and carrots and bring to a boil. Reduce heat to low, cover and simmer for one hour, or until vegetables are tender.

Step 4

Add the green beans, peas and beans and allow to heat through, about 15 minutes. Finally add the chopped parsley and season with salt and pepper to taste.

Nutrition Facts

Per Serving: 133 calories; protein 5.7g; carbohydrates 25.1g; fat 2g; cholesterol 3.8mg; sodium 314.2mg.

Kitchen Sink Soup
Recipe Summary

Prep: 20 mins

Cook: 30 mins

Total: 50 mins

Servings: 10

Yield: 10 servings

Ingredients

- 10 cups chicken broth
- 2 potatoes, cubed
- 2 carrots, sliced
- 2 stalks celery, diced
- 5 fresh mushrooms, sliced
- 1 green bell pepper, chopped
- 1 fresh broccoli, chopped
- 4 cups cauliflower florets
- 1 parsnip, sliced
- 1 onion, chopped
- 1 cup green peas
- 1 cup cut green beans, drained
- 1 cup wax beans, drained

- ½ cup cooked chickpeas
- ½ cup cooked navy beans
- salt and pepper to taste
- 1 teaspoon dried parsley

Directions

Step 1

In a large stockpot, combine all the ingredients and cook over medium heat partially covered for about 30 minutes or until all the vegetables are tender. Serve hot with buttered biscuits.

Nutrition Facts

Per Serving: 160 calories; protein 10.3g; carbohydrates 26.3g; fat 1.9g; sodium 1008.1mg.

Chocolate Chip Cookies for Special Diets

Recipe Summary

Prep: 15 mins

Cook: 12 mins

Additional: 23 mins

Total: 50 mins

Servings: 48

Yield: 4 dozen

Ingredients

- ½ cup butter, softened
- ¾ cup granulated artificial sweetener
- 2 tablespoons water
- ½ teaspoon vanilla extract
- 1 egg, beaten
- 1 ⅛ cups all-purpose flour
- ½ teaspoon baking soda
- ½ teaspoon salt
- ½ cup semisweet chocolate chips
- ½ cup chopped pecans

Directions

Step 1

Preheat oven to 375 degrees F (190 degrees C).

Step 2

In a medium bowl, cream together the butter and sugar substitute. Mix in water, vanilla, and egg. Sift together the flour, baking soda, and salt; stir into the creamed mixture. Mix in the chocolate chips and pecans. Drop cookies by heaping teaspoonfuls onto a cookie sheet.

Step 3

Bake in the preheated oven for 10 to 12 minutes. Remove from cookie sheets to cool on wire racks. These cookies freeze well.

Nutrition Facts

Per Serving: 60 calories; protein 4.2g; carbohydrates 3.5g; fat 3.4g; cholesterol 9mg; sodium 53.8mg.

Gluten-Free Chocolate Chip Cookies

Recipe Summary

Prep: 15 mins

Cook: 10 mins

Additional: 10 mins

Total: 35 mins

Servings: 24

Yield: 2 dozen

Ingredients

- ½ cup coconut palm sugar
- ¼ cup extra-virgin coconut oil, at room temperature
- ½ teaspoon baking soda
- Himalayan pink salt to taste
- 2 cups almond flour
- 2 eggs
- 1 tablespoon vanilla extract
- 1 cup chocolate chips (such as Ghirardelli®)

Directions

Step 1

Preheat oven to 350 degrees F (175 degrees C). Lightly grease a baking sheet.

Step 2

Combine coconut sugar, coconut oil, baking soda, and salt in a large bowl; beat with a handheld electric mixer until smooth. Add almond flour, eggs, and vanilla extract. Beat dough at medium speed, scraping the bottom and sides of the bowl, until well mixed, about 1 minute.

Step 3

Fold chocolate chips into the dough. Grease your palms lightly with coconut oil; drop tablespoonfuls of dough onto the baking sheet.

Step 4

Bake in the preheated oven until golden brown, 10 to 12 minutes. Let cool on the baking sheet, about 10 minutes.

Nutrition Facts

Per Serving: 139 calories; protein 3g; carbohydrates 11.2g; fat 9.9g; cholesterol 15.5mg; sodium 36.2mg.

CONCLUSION

The MIND Diet consists of 15 dietary components, including 10 "brain-healthy food groups" and five "unhealthy-brain" food groups. The healthy groups include berries, green leafy vegetables as well as other vegetables, whole grains, nuts, beans, fish, poultry, olive oil and wine. The unhealthy groups are red meats, butter and stick margarine, cheese, pastries and sweets, and fried or fast food. What's more interesting is that the MIND Diet is easier to follow than the Mediterranean Diet, which calls for daily consumption of fish and three to four servings of both fruits and vegetables, Morris says. And where the Mediterranean and DASH diet plans promote fruit intake in general, berries are the only recommended fruit as part of the MIND Diet. "Blueberries are one of the more potent foods in terms of protecting the brain, "says Morris, and strawberries have also performed well in past studies examining the effects of food on cognitive function.

MIND Diet study indicate strong preliminary evidence that brain-boosting benefits can be found in food intake and diet regimens. More importantly, we now have clear evidence of the fact that the early adoption of new "brain healthy" eating habits, even in moderation, can boost brain and lessen the risks of cognitive decline. The MIND diet is designed to prevent dementia and loss of brain function as you age. It combines the Mediterranean diet and the DASH diet to create a dietary pattern that focuses specifically on brain health.

www.ingramcontent.com/pod-product-compliance
Lightning Source LLC
Chambersburg PA
CBHW071338130726
47996CB00002B/789